Modern Dental Thermoforming

The Highly Profitable Path to Clinical Excellence, Consistency and Precision

© Copyright 2009 Good Innovations Pty Limited

All rights reserved
No part of this publication may be reproduced,
stored in a retrieval system or transmitted without written permission.

ISBN 978-0-9578929-2-7 (PDF Version)
ISBN 978-0-9578929-3-4 (Print Version)

1. Medical Science – Dentistry 2. Sports & Games 3. Education 4. Sports Safety

A catalogue record for this publication is
available from the National Library of Australia

Good Innovations publications may be purchased for educational,
business or sales promotional use.
For more information please email: info@mouthguardsafety.com
or write:
Good Innovations Pty Ltd,
80 Avalon Parade, Avalon, NSW 2107, Australia

Produced by

Good Innovations

www.goodinnovations.com

I0031527

About the Author

Julian Hodges has more than 25 years experience of thermoforming and as such he is a recognized world leader and sought after international advisor. He has spoken, published and consulted to acclaim in Europe, Asia and the United States. He has advised sports people, sporting associations, dentists, universities, colleges, the military and dental laboratories including the world's largest.

Julian has been described as, *"Unique in his field"* and, *"A Coach that achieves outstanding results."*

His great skill has been to lift the knowledge of thermoforming, the level of comfort and the techniques to make thermoformed appliances to a continually higher level. He presents, what can be a complex subject, in a simple, balanced, practical way that can be immediately and easily understood and implemented.

Julian held the world's first courses to teach custom laminating techniques and is credited, with proving the necessity for mouthguard standards.

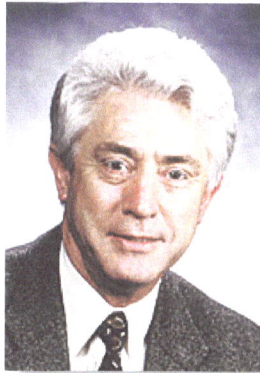

Disclaimer

The selection and use of thermoforming equipment, materials and accessories is always a matter for specialist professional assessment for each application.

The content and commentary within this manual is by way of general guideline only. It is not intended as any substitution for qualified, specialist dental or medical advice. The information is not provided with the intention of giving a comprehensive understanding of the way in which products will perform or their suitability for any use in any particular circumstance.

The information herein is not held out as to accuracy, specifically or generally.

Contents – Modern Dental Thermoforming

A New, Highly Profitable Path to Clinical Excellence, Consistency and Precision

Discover a Paradigm Shift in the Range and Profitability of Thermoforming with an Occludator Attachment

Replicating a construction bite with zero additional minutes of thermoforming time

Thermoforming Basics

13 Important Points That Will Instantly Improve Your Thermoforming Results

Why the Materials you Buy May Significantly Affect your Clinical Results

Save Time and Make Life Easier with the Right Instruments and Accessories

Conclusion – Turn Knowledge into Action and Reap the Benefits

Bonus Tools to Eliminate Risk and Reach the Right Decision

Thermoforming Profit Calculator

Annual Profit from a System, Annual Return on Investment, Number of Months to Recover Your Investment

Scorecards to Rate and Identify the Best System for You

Will the System You are Considering Really Produce The Result You Need?

Vacuum Systems, Pressure Systems

Note: If you have purchased a printed copy of Modern Dental Thermoforming and would like the **bonus tools**, please email info@mouthguardsafety.com. You will need to include your purchase order details in the email.

Foreward and Executive Summary

Modern Dental Thermoforming – A New, Highly Profitable Path to Clinical Excellence, Consistency and Precision

The sole purpose of this resource for Dental Professionals is to provide knowledge and know-how so that balanced, sound decisions may be made in the financial, clinical and operational assessment of thermoforming systems.

Modern Dental Thermoforming closely describes and analyses the surprising profits, range of applications, benefits and opportunities of modern dental thermoforming together with the pitfalls, limitations and misconceptions. The net result is; you will be in a position to decide if a thermoforming system is appropriate for your practice or laboratory and if so, just what you can reasonably expect it to deliver, clinically and financially.

Modern Dental Thermoforming is based on the accumulated knowledge and experience I have gained in 25+ years of coaching, advising, trouble-shooting and marketing thermoforming at the highest levels. I have no financial links with any thermoforming equipment or material producer.

The Unrealised Potential and Profitability of Thermoforming

Whether or not your knowledge and experience of thermoforming is elementary, or you have experienced dubious thermoforming outcomes, *Modern Dental Thermoforming* will show you a new, financially viable path to thermoforming clinical excellence, consistency and precision.

You will know as much as the experts. Skills will easily be developed with the right equipment, materials, instruments and accessories. You will produce appliances that are highly comfortable and usually a noticeable improvement on those produced by traditional methods.

Expect to:

- Build comfortable, crystal clear, highly polished, hard or soft/hard splints that fit with a balanced occlusal plane and point contact in 15 to 20 minutes
- Easily and simply add ramps, cuspid guidance or any other features to splints with such precision and control they are indistinguishable from processed splints
- Form and finish micron accurate bleaching trays in a few minutes
- Provide unparalleled levels of protection with state of the art, multi-layer sports mouthguards and softer, comfortable, fun mouthguards with graphics for kids
- Build comfortable interim partial dentures for implant patients in 25 to 35 minutes

- Reduce by 85% the free monomers of ortho devices made by the traditional 'salt and pepper' technique

Bonus Tools to Minimise Risk

Every dental professional knows there are potential problems and associated risks with any investment. Identifying risk is a consistent theme throughout *Modern Dental Thermoforming*. Potential problems are highlighted rather than glossed over or ignored.

A free Bonus Report and two Interactive Tools are unique resources that allow you to step back and realistically evaluate the advantages and the problems of thermoforming.

Thermoforming Profit Calculator is another interactive tool. Enter elementary data such as lab fees and material costs and it will calculate the profit, return on investment and the number of months it will take to get your money back.

Risk Reduction Scorecards are an interactive tool to rate and identify the most appropriate thermoforming systems for you. The *Scorecards* identify the major features of vacuum and pressure systems, allowing you to rate and compare competing brands and models to reach a clear, unequivocal result.

With these tools and the extensive information available for the first time in *Modern Dental Thermoforming,* you will be able to comfortably make balanced, informed decisions that are in your best interests and those of your patients and clients.

I wish you every success

Julian Hodges
Avalon Beach, Sydney, Australia
April 2009

Note: If you have purchased a printed copy of Modern Dental Thermoforming and would like the bonus tools, please email info@mouthguardsafety.com. You will need to include your purchase order details in the email.

The Benefits you Should Demand from a Thermoforming System

As clinical demands and patient expectation grow in dentistry, patient's experiences and comfort dramatically affect the success of practices. Due to its accuracy, thermoformed devices produced with a good system and high quality materials, bring great patient praise and referrals.

These are some of the benefits you should expect by investing in one of today's better thermoforming systems:

Financial Viability

- 100% return on your investment (ROI) in less than a year. Many installations achieve up to 400% return in Year 1.
- Use the FREE 'Thermoforming Profit Calculator' supplied with this manual. Insert the data specific to your practice or laboratory to calculate:
  - Annual profit a system will generate for you
  - The Return on Investment
  - Number of months it will take to recover your investment

Production

- Simple, fast, easy training produces high quality results
- Devices can be produced with general practice staff and are not dependent on high skill levels
- Saves time – 15 minute occlusal splints
- Lower administration complexity and costs
- Elimination of or at least a massive reduction in free monomers. For example, orthodontic expansion plates may have up to 85% reduction in free monomers over the 'salt and pepper' technique
- Minimal or zero noise levels

Clinical

- More treatment options
  - Increases revenue
  - Improves patient experience

- Micron accurate adaptation
  - Gives consistency
  - Reduces chair time for patient and doctor
  - Improves device retention
  - Reduces remakes with 'first time every time fit'
  - Gives greater comfort
- Improved clinical results
  - Patients wear devices longer
  - Patients are more compliant and more willing to follow instructions

Laboratories

- Advanced thermoforming systems increase the number of revenue streams, the lab's service to clients and the quality and acceptability of its output

Thirty-Seven Applications that Lift the Quality of Dentistry

In most practices or laboratories, thermoforming machines are usually used for a small range of appliances. There is little doubt however, when you or your staff have discovered how easy it is to achieve superlative clinical results, you and they will want to apply thermoforming techniques to an ever-increasing range of applications.

Although not all machines can be used to produce the entire range of thermoformed devices, the better the system, the greater the number of devices it will produce.

It is difficult if not impossible to predict all the future applications of thermoforming you will need. Therefore, invest in a machine that will allow you to do more than you currently imagine necessary.

These are the applications that currently can be easily, accurately and quickly produced with a well designed thermoforming machine and high quality materials:

Splints

- Nightguards
- Hard Occlusal Splints
- Soft/Hard Occlusal Splints (Talon type)
- Semi-Hard Monomer-Free Occlusal Splints with 95 Shore A Hardness
- Bruxism Splints
- Stress Release Splints
- Stabilization Splints
- Jaw Fracture Splints

Cosmetic Dentistry

- Bleaching Trays
- Temporary Crowns and Bridges
- Tooth Jewellery Matrices

Mouthguards

- Single layer Mouthguards
- Custom Laminated Mouthguards (Type 3)

- Custom Laminated Mouthguards with a Hard Bonded Layer
- Orthodontic Mouthguards – for example, with lingual reinforcing

Implants

- Drilling Templates
- Orientation Splints
- Interim Partial Dentures

Trays

- Impression Trays
- Fluoride Trays
- Medication Trays
- Gingival Dressings
- Surgical Bandages

Orthodontics

- Retainers (Essix type)
- Expansion Plates
- Bracket Transfer Trays for Indirect Bonding
- Etching Masks for Bracket Transfer
- Positioners
- Other Orthodontic Appliances and Gnatho-Orthopaedic aids such as Skeletal Retainers

Anti Snoring and Sleep Apnoea Devices

Laboratory

- Model Duplication
- Crown and Bridge Copings
- Denture Base Plates
- Bite Plates
- Denture Repairs
- Model Protection

Radiology and Radiotherapy

- Protection Splints

How to Avoid Purchasing a Thermoforming Dinosaur

Creating the Foundation for Outstanding Results

Equipment is the foundation of thermoforming. You can change materials and modify techniques, but once you have chosen the equipment, you are locked in. You have put into place a platform for excellence and progress or, a clinical millstone and a financial straight jacket that will probably remain with you for many years.

It is **vitally** important to invest in the equipment that will do the job you **really need** it to do! Carefully calculate the financial return and you will usually find it is greater than expected, allowing you to install a machine that suits you best rather than compromising and being left with a more costly device that does not meet your standards or the needs of your patients.

There are 5 types of thermoforming machines and many brands. They can be:

- Difficult or simple and easy to use
- Costly or economic
- Time consuming to use or efficient and highly productive
- Limited or have wide ranging application, and
- Give poor, indifferent adaptation or provide micron accurate results

For today's dentistry the only types of machine you should consider are PRESSURE or RAPID HIGH VACUUM.

Pressure Machines Apply More Forming Power

Pressure machines are the benchmark by which the precision of all thermoforming is judged.

- Pressure machines normally operate between 60 to 80 psi (4.2 to 5.7 kg/cm^2) and deliver 10 to 15 times more forming power than old square low-vacuum machines.
- As the forming power pressure of machines is applied above the foil, materials are pushed towards the gingiva and sulcus causing a clinically preferable wall taper.
- Pressure machines are particularly suitable for high output laboratories. They may require a higher level of operator skill.
- Pressure machines may be used for all thermoformed appliances and especially for custom laminated mouthguards with graphics and a clear outer layer (fewer air inclusions).

- If you intend to develop a serious mouthguard business, particularly with the more protective custom laminated designs, install a pressure machine. Be careful! Some pressure machines are more suitable than others for mouthguard production.
- If you intend to produce splints, denture repairs, orthodontic and snoring and sleep apnoea devices that require self cure acrylics, consider a pressure machine that has an optional polymerisation flask. By using high pressure to suppress the boiling point of the monomer, the quality of clear self cure acrylics is first class.

Why Rapid High-Vacuum Reservoir Machines are Ideal for Most Practices

Rapid High-Vacuum Reservoir Machines can produce outstanding results and provide the best combination of features for most dental practices. An internal pump **creates a vacuum as the foil is heating**. When the heated foil is sealed over the model the vacuum is instantaneously and aggressively released with results that often are **difficult to distinguish from pressure**.

- Machines of this type should achieve an 80% vacuum
- They should be able to adapt all thermoforming materials up to 6.0 mm (0.25 inches) thick
- Functions can be electronically controlled
- With little training they are simple and easy to use by most dental office staff

Occludators

A rapid high-vacuum machine, fitted with an Occludator transforms the thermoforming process and *must be seriously considered* whenever there is a possibility that occlusal splints may be required. Read, *Discover A Paradigm Shift In The Range And Profitability Of Thermoforming With An Interfaced Occludator*.

Note: Where absolute precision is required, for example with implant stents, check the precision you require by comparing the degree of adaptation with the results from a pressure machine and with the materials you will use in practice.

Compressed Air Ejector Machines

First invented in the very early 1980's these machines use a compressed air venturi to create an instant vacuum. Simple devices such as Bleaching Stents can be produced and a limited range of mouthguards may be laminated.

Vacuum Reservoir machines produce superior results.

Square Motor Driven Low Vacuum Machines

Square Motor Driven Low Vacuum Machines are dental dinosaurs. Why are they still used? They are cheap!! Purchasers may not realise what can be achieved with superior technology and may not be aware clinical standards are being compromised.

They have an overhead radiant heater and usually adapt square materials by activating a vacuum pump once the foil has been heated. Designed 50 years ago, their level of adaptation is no longer acceptable. These machines show their age:

- Forming power is low
- The standard of adaptation is being increasingly criticised
- They are noisy
- Adaptation varies
- The radiant heaters are fierce and inconsistent
- It is virtually impossible to laminate mouthguards and,
- They are limited in their application

Rubber Dam/Venturi Systems

Apart from flasking and packing or adapting by hand, Rubber Dam/Venturi Systems are the oldest in use. They are linked to a water tap or a vacuum source.

Materials are usually softened in water so the high heat that is essential for precise adaptation cannot be used. Definition is low. Their popularity is understandably declining.

Some operators claim better results can be obtained with venturi systems than low vacuum machines.

Why it is Essential to Have Full Forming Power Before the Completion of the Heating Cycle

There are two essential aspects to forming power:

- First and most important is; *forming power must be fast and aggressive*
- Secondly; the total amount of forming power must be sufficient

High speed adaptation is vital which is why commercial dental laboratories and specialist practices that need highly accurate appliances have used pressure machines for so long. However, even a pressure machine cannot produce a high level of adaptation if the adapting force is applied too slowly. Let me explain:

If you are forming with a pressure machine and do not switch on the compressor until *after* the foil had been heated the results must be poor because, by the time the compressor has built up sufficient pressure, the foil will be cold and unable to be formed.

Therefore full forming power has to be immediately available and, to do that, *forming power must be created before the heating cycle is completed.*

The older square low-vacuum machines have limited precision because of the slow build up of forming power. This is what happens. These machines may make a lot of noise but the motor is not activated until the foil is hot. A vacuum is only being created therefore during the forming process, and that is too slow! The foil comes in contact with the centrals and it is then dragged from the incisal points. The material becomes thin and inconsistent in thickness.

With fast, aggressive forming power the material is attacked and is wrapped or thrust into place with far less stretching or distortion.

The absolute rule for precision and consistent results is:

*Full Forming Power **Must** Be Immediately Available at the Completion The Completion Of The Heating Cycle!!*
The Sudden Release Of Forming Power Gives Aggressive, Fast Adaptation And Micron Accurate Results.

This is where pressure machines excel over vacuum. Rapid high-vacuum machines produce excellent results for most appliances but, they may not have the precision you require in all applications.

Before you buy a machine, check it will produce the devices you require to the standard you want and with the materials you will use.

What you Need to Know About Heating – If you are Serious About Achieving First Class Results

Having the correct heating system is fundamental to efficient, clinically excellent thermoformed devices. Substandard heating systems may cause insurmountable difficulties when producing accurate, comfortable, durable and correctly functioning appliances.

The Best Heating for Dental Thermoforming

Infrared is the best type of heat for thermoforming; it produces an <u>even</u> heat that <u>penetrates</u> the foil with less risk of damaging or changing the physical properties of thermoforming materials.

Medium wave infra-red is the most widely used but it requires a separate warm-up phase unless the heater has electronic temperature control as opposed to time control.

For instantaneous heat use a short wave infra-red system. However, to avoid damaging materials, short wave systems require precise controls such as those developed and patented by Scheu Dental.

With halogen heating, which also provides instant heat, check occupational health and safety requirements because there are recommendations that sunglasses should be used to protect against emission from some halogen heaters.

Why You Will Always Get Poor Results from Radiant Heaters

The radiant heaters of the older square low-vacuum machines have the solitary advantage of being cheap. But the *poorest* thermoforming results are from the cruder, radiant, toaster type heaters usually found on these machines. These heaters may be great for toast but, by today's standards, they are not good for even moderate quality dental thermoforming.

Have you experienced these negative features?

- Hot and cold spots giving inconsistent heat across the foil
- One surface of the foil being fiercely heated, (sometimes altering its molecular structure and damaging the foil), leaving the fitting surface cold. The result? Accuracy will be poor because the cool side is adapted to the model and is not heated through. Your appliances will inevitably reflect this
- Difficulty obtaining the heat penetration that is necessary to custom laminate mouthguards

Which Is Better? To Heat the Fitting or Non-Fitting Surface of the Foil

Some manufacturers state that to improve adaptation it is better to heat the fitting surface of a foil because the surface temperature may be 60°C higher.

Whilst there is some validity in this statement and, depending upon the application and the type of material being heated, the benefits are questionable when compared to applying infrared heat to the side of the foil that does not contact the model. The reasons are:

- Better results with Hard/Soft (Talon type) Splints: The hard material has a higher melting point and therefore should be heated first. In this way the hard material has the correct consistency and will not force out the softer material when the foil is formed. *The result is better fitting, more durable splints*
- Greater patient comfort: Materials shrink and tighten up when cooling. Therefore, if the coolest side of the foil is presented to the model there will be less cooling shrinkage and consequently more patient comfort especially with hard splint materials
- Many of the best splint materials have a thin polyethylene insulation foil to act as a spacer and produce a crystal clear finish. These foils ensure that fine particles or thermoforming granules are not imbedded into the splint. It is not possible to have the benefits of insulating foils when they are destroyed by higher and fiercer direct heat to the foil's fitting surface
- For some it is easier to make custom laminated mouthguards
- There is better adaptation of laboratory copings

Discover a Paradigm Shift in the Range and Profitability of Thermoforming with an Occludator Attachment

Replicating a construction bite with zero additional minutes of thermoforming time

Dr Hans Peter Kopp who, incidentally, invented rapid high-vacuum systems, created a paradigm shift in the profitability, range and ease of use of thermoforming by attaching an Occludator to a rapid high vacuum thermoforming machine.

By being able to impose an imprint of an opposing arch into softened thermoformed material without the need for additional production time, the thermoforming process for splints, mouthguards and positioners is transformed.

Staff quickly achieve fast first class results even with little previous experience. For instance:

- In 15 minutes a reasonably skilled operator can produce a hard, clear, highly polished splint with a polished occlusal plane and point contact. (Placing a 1.0 mm or 1.5 mm polyethylene foil between the formed splint and its opposing arch creates a flat occlusal plane.) The foil is then removed and whilst the splint is warm and pliable, the contact points are registered.
- In mouthguard production, a complete and time consuming step can be eliminated by creating an opposing bite in the guard.

Note: Occludators can only be realistically used with Rapid High Vacuum machines. They cannot be used with pressure machines where the model is contained within the pressure chamber.

New Occudator Design Replicates the Rotational Measurements of Average Movement Articulators

Dr Kopp's original design required the use a construction bite to avoid variations between the vertical dimensions of an Occludator and an average movement articulator.

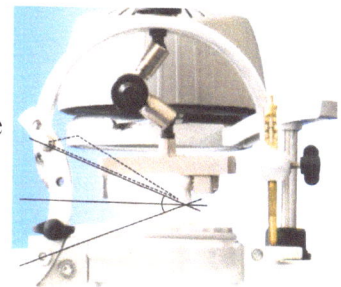

The most recent design has overcome this restriction. The rotational measurements of the Occluform-3 reflect those of an average movement articulator, greatly assisting the production of mouthguards and splints. It has a Bonwill triangle with a side length of 11.5cm (indicated by the dashed triangle) and a Balkwill angle of 20°.

Thermoforming Basics

13 Important Points That Will Instantly Improve Your Thermoforming Results

1. During thermoforming, materials stretch and become thinner. Generally they thin by approximately 20% with each 1.0 cm (0.4 inch) of model height. It is therefore advantageous to embed models in granules so that only the required area is thermoformed

2. Models should be poured with Type III stone or better (not plaster) and can be slightly damp

3. Plastic or varnished models are impermeable to air and may cause incomplete adaptation because air cannot be pushed into the model

4. Model bases should be trimmed flat

5. Set up the models so that labial surfaces of the centrals are perpendicular

6. To obtain consistent thickness over the whole model, foils should be presented perpendicular to the model and not at an angle

7. All models can break when hard materials are removed after thermoforming. The use of a super-hard stone will not solve the problem. It is better to work with a duplicate model

8. Tension across the dental arch caused with hard splint materials, is reduced by heating the non-fitting surface of the foil

9. The final thermoforming action occurs when the foil is allowed to cool and therefore to shrink onto the model. This is especially important when forming hard thick foils, possibly 5.0 mm thick with a vacuum machine and where there are few, if any, undercuts

10. Ensure all materials are physiologically listed by the Health Authorities as harmless and hypoallergenic

11. Do not remove the high shine from the highly polished surfaces of formed materials unless there is no alternative. You will only have to spend time replacing the high shine and the results you obtain are unlikely to be as good as the original

12. Cutting, finishing and polishing thermoformable materials may require technique changes. Avoid creating heat with high speeds and high-pressure. The appliance may deform and burs can become clogged, decreasing their efficiency

13. **Do not just buy a machine, set up a System** – that is the Equipment, Instruments, Materials and Accessories

Why the Materials you Buy May Significantly Affect your Clinical Results

Is it possible to purchase a good thermoforming machine and still have an unsatisfactory result? YES! There are vast differences in the quality of materials available to you. Some are good – many are bad.

We now know the equipment features that are required to provide a foundation and a springboard for great thermoforming. There is no doubt that good equipment will markedly improve your results. But, achieving a great result does not depend solely on the equipment you select.

Materials too can seriously affect the forming process by cooling quickly (e.g. with thin foils and fast cooling polymers such as polyethylene). Mouthguard materials retain heat while others distort with slow adaptation.

Don't Let Someone Sell you a Problem

The best materials are easier to use and are more stable. They usually cost a little more.

The worst materials are hard to adapt, inconsistent and technique critical. They are invariably on 'Special Offer' and are cheap but they can cost you a fortune in lost time, remakes, staff confusion and patient disappointment. For example, one of the troubles with bleaching trays is that the manufacturers of bleaching agents have a great interest in bleaching agents but possibly little knowledge or indeed, interest in the quality of tray materials. In the dollar driven search for cheaper and cheaper materials they may not fully understand the need for high quality materials.

For appliances with more consistency in their thickness and greater comfort, durability and protection, use a material that will achieve this without compromise.

Look for these features:

- Materials that do not bubble or distort in the heating process.
- Hard or Soft/Hard splint materials that have a fine (0.1 mm) separating foil to create a pressure release for patients and give a crystal clear finish. During the thermoforming process micro-fine dust particles can be imbedded in the splint material.
- Splint and ortho materials that bond well with cold cure acrylics.

The Secrets About Mouthguard Materials That Others Can't or Won't Tell You

This excerpt from Mouthguard Mastery features how to make the most protective mouthguards ever tested. It will give you an insight into what can happen to thermoforming materials and how to look for flaws.

There are many mouthguard materials. They vary in quality and price. So how can you <u>instantly</u> know if the material you are being offered is the quality you need?

Have you ever wondered why some materials go <u>thick and thin</u> when you heat them?

Have you ever wondered why some materials get <u>harder</u> or <u>change</u> their physical properties when you have formed them?

And have you wondered why your mouthguards are <u>too thin</u>?

In the majority of cases it is **not your fault**. It's just that the manufacturer did not give you the materials you needed.

It is difficult for you to assess mouthguard materials because there are no standards and so few people know about them.

The answer to these questions is:

Don't Let Someone <u>Sell</u> You a Problem!

Mouthguard materials go thick and thin when you heat them because of **inconsistencies** in the materials. They are <u>not</u> homogeneous!

How can <u>you</u> check for non-homogeneity?

- Look at the surface of the foil. If it is not <u>completely</u> smooth and has processing marks the foil probably has a memory and will recover when you heat it.
- An easy way to check a translucent foil is. Hold it up to a light and, if you can see inconsistency and the material is not totally homogenous, it will have an in built memory.
- Next, from side on, check the thickness of the foil. If it varies, then the results you get will vary. That's virtually guaranteed.

Variations in thickness and the consistency of mouthguard materials are a result of <u>poor</u> quality control or production methods. In any event, the manufacturer is saving money and **passing the problem on to you!**

Easy to Use Materials Will Save You Time and Money and Reduce Your Remakes

When the physical properties of mouthguard materials change in the heating and adaptation process, it is because the manufacturer is probably again saving money at your and your patients' expense.

One reason is that the materials are <u>not dense</u> enough. This reduces the manufacturer's raw material costs. But, it means that these materials **compact** with heat and forming pressure. They become thinner and sometimes harder.

Another reason is that the manufacturer may use <u>low-grade</u> base stock or a high proportion of <u>recycled material</u>. Sometimes both!

Check that the materials you buy have clarity and vibrancy. As in life, things that are dull and lifeless are a warning sign! Mouthguard materials are no different!

Where are the Best Sources for Dependable High Quality Thermoforming Materials?

The best thermoforming materials all currently come from the main German manufacturers: *Erkodent, Scheu and Dreve*.

Save Time and Make Life Easier with the Right Instruments and Accessories

The labour cost of thermoforming is ultimately far greater than the machine cost and therefore, irrespective of how good your thermoformer may be, specific attention should be paid to using the right instruments and accessories because they can literally cut production time in half. It is here the best operators shine.

Fortunately the top manufacturers have developed complete systems to reduce the technical demands and make thermoforming easier, stress-free and more profitable.

Keep it Simple!

Select instruments that can be used on hard as well as soft materials, that way the number of instruments you may need will be halved.

Rotating Instruments

No more than 5 carefully chosen burs and discs are usually needed for all thermoforming applications.

Fast Cutting Burs

Fissure burs with a counter-rotational spiral give a fast, clean finish, saving time. Use at a fast cutting speed of up to 25,000 rpm.

Precise Contouring

Fine steel milling 0.8 mm to 1.0 mm twist drills produce remarkable results and stunning precision. Use these burs at 25,000 rpm and let the bur do the work – just guide it, gently, if you don't it will break.

Note: This is a cutting bur, not a trimming bur. For the bur to work always leave sufficient material from the initial cut out from the foil.

Trimming

Use a fine cross cut cone shaped tungsten carbide for fast, clean, smooth trimming. The point gives easy access to confined interproximal spaces.
A pear shaped fine crosscut tungsten carbide bur is better for occlusal surfaces.

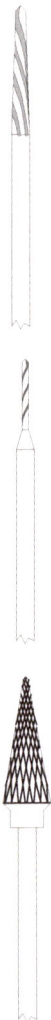

Note: Use low rpm's to avoid generating heat which causes hot material to clog the cutting area of the bur, reducing its efficiency.

Finishing

Look for a soft, flexible disc that has a stabilised but open structure, which reduces heat generation. Use discs at low speeds – 4,000 to 10,000 rpm.

Silicone points are an alternative although not as efficient.

Polishing

Do not remove the high shine from the highly polished surfaces of formed materials unless there is no alternative. You will only have to spend time restoring the high shine. Your best results may not be as good as the original.

For mouthguard materials a spectacular high shine can be obtained with a butane powered Hot Air Pen with a 3 mm to 4 mm (0.12 - 0.16 inch) nozzle. This also requires the use of high quality materials.

Linen/cotton polishing discs with traditional polishing mediums are best for hard materials.

Note: Too much pressure when using a polishing lathe will generate heat and distort the appliance.

Remember: If you contour and trim accurately and finish with care, many thermoformed appliances will not require further polishing

Scissors – The Right Scissors Save Time

Find the correct scissors and you will be surprised at just how effective they are. With well designed scissors you will avoid the tedium and hazards of cutting out soft foils and thinner hard foils with a hot knife or scalpel and save time when using burs.

I recommend scissors with curved slip resistant blades, a blade length of 35 mm to 50 mm (2 inches) and an overall length 100 mm to 125 mm (4.0 to 5.0 inches). You will be surprised just how thick a foil they will easily cut through.

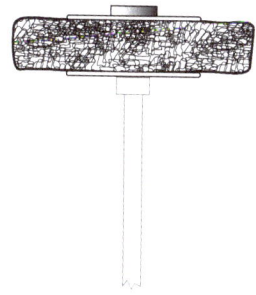

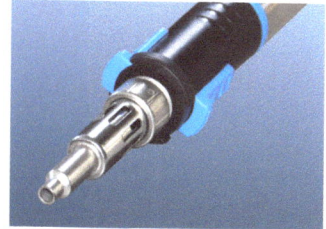

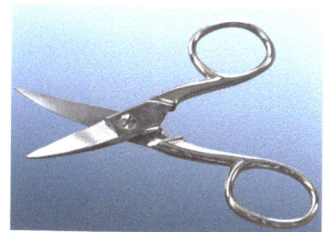

Granules – Make Thermoforming Easier and Improve Results

Granules save time and give you greater control in the thermoforming process. Granules have not been universally popular in the past simply because of perceived handing difficulties. Now the better machines are designed so you can have all the benefits of using granules and handling is simple.

Use granules to:

- Limit model height – reduces thinning of the foil
- Setting the model up in the correct position and at the correct angle – faster and easier than using a model trimmer; reduces anterior thinning
- Blocking out – easier removable of model from the formed foil; controls material thickness; saves models

Notes:

- Use a separator foil when forming with soft materials (Check the heating system of the machine will allow this)
- Look for a machine that makes handling granules simple
- Use granules designed for thermoforming; you have more control, a better result and a faster set up. Substituting lead shot or rice will ultimately be more expensive, contaminate the foil and may result in the untimely demise of your machine.
- Use a magnet to round up wayward granules

Cold Cure Resins – Allow the Production of Any Splint Design

With the right cold cure resin and good thermoforming materials you will be able to produce any splint design you need – quickly and surprisingly easily.

For many years I was under the illusion that it was not possible to add cold cure to formed splint material. Then the penny dropped! Most cold cures have fast working times and high shrinkage values, which are ideal for ortho appliances but not for thermoforming. The opposite is needed!

- Long working time. Allows the cold cure to be placed and adjusted with adequate working time and without the need for dams. It significantly reduces post cure adjustment and finishing. Look for a cold cure with 6 to 8 minutes working time
- Low shrinkage values. With high shrinkage acrylics the bond between the cold cure and the formed material is compromised in the polymerisation process. This is particular noticeable at featheredge margins. Minimal shrinkage cold cures eliminate this problem.

Tips:

- Release the surface tension on the formed base – remove the splint from the model and apply monomer to those areas to which acrylic will be added
- Allow extended working time cold cures to reach a soft putty-like state before applying to the base
- Apply monomer to the feather edge at the join of the formed base and cold cure

Polymerisation Flasks

The high 4 to 6 Bar pressure of some pressure machines makes them ideal for polymerising acrylics. The high pressure suppresses the boiling point of the monomer to give bubble-free and higher quality results.

Polymerisation flasks for pressure thermoforming machines do not have pressure gauges or sealing rings to malfunction and leak. Only the job needs to be covered by water.

Polymerisation flasks in pressure machines are excellent for:

- Splints
- Denture repairs
- Orthodontic appliances
- Snoring and sleep apnoea devices

Conclusion – Turn Knowledge into Action and Reap the Benefits

You now have an extensive understanding of thermoforming, its function, impact and its remarkable potential for improved clinical, organisational and financial rewards. You have an understanding too, of features to avoid and the associated risks. You know as much, if not more than most 'experts'.

At what point do you turn your new knowledge into action so you gain all the benefits of thermoforming? One way is to **place a premium on getting things done**. To do that you can use to great advantage, the unique interactive *Profit Calculator* and the *Risk Reduction Scorecard* to clearly identify whether or not investing in a thermoforming system is appropriate for business or practice.

The time of reading, discussing and thinking about thermoforming is over. It is now up to you. The time has arrived to turn your new knowledge into a decision and that decision into action.

I am keenly aware it is not the money you spent purchasing this manual that is most important, because it can be replaced: but it is the investment of your time in reading it which cannot be replaced. For this reason I thank you for your trust and sincerely hope that it has been thoroughly worth your while.

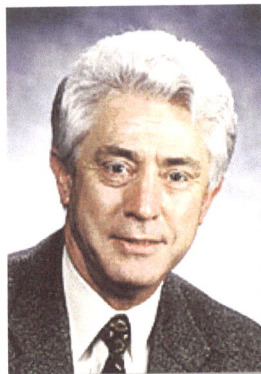

Julian Hodges
Avalon, Australia
April 2009